Yoga

4-Week Step By Step Guide for Yoga Beginners. Become A Yoga Guru Of Your Own Physical, Mental And Spiritual Self

Jill Hesson

Table of Contents

Introduction 1

The Basics..2

Why Practice Yoga?...3

How to Adopt Yoga in 4 weeks: A Three Step Approach 7

    Step 1: Calm Down 7

    Step 2: Focus On Your Breath......................................8

    Step 3: Start With Basic Postures 9

Week One 10

    Warm-Up Exercises 10

    Standing Asanas 16

    4: Half-Moon Pose 20

Week Two...21

    Seated and Kneeling Asanas 21

Week Three 26

    Supine & Prone Asanas 26

    Twists Asanas 30

    14: Low Lunge Twist... 33

Week Four 34

    Inverted and Balance Asana.. 34

Conclusion... 40

Introduction

I want to thank you and congratulate you for downloading the book, *"Yoga: 4-Week Step By Step Guide for Yoga Beginners. Become A Yoga Guru Of Your Own Physical, Mental And Spiritual Self"*.

This book has actionable information that will help you to become a yoga guru of your physical, mental and spiritual self in as little as 4 weeks.

We live in a world where we feel completely lost and just riding along. We feel as if we just exist without any particular purpose in life. When that happens, anxiousness, stress and depression starts creeping in, and we stop taking care of how we look as well as our health. The result is an unhealthy lifestyle, which may even advance to various health complications. Have you gotten to that point of your life where you feel you need to find your purpose and bring order to your currently disorderly life?

Well, yoga can do all that since it can help you to bring the much needed order in your physical, mental and spiritual life. What do you think yoga is? Do you think of it as simply executing Olympics level gymnastics stunts? Well, yoga is much more than these stunts. This book will introduce you to yoga, what it is all about and how you can start practicing yoga in as little as 4 weeks.

Thanks again for downloading this book. I hope you enjoy it!

The Basics

What is yoga?

"*Yoga*" is a Sanskrit word formed from a Latin word '*yoke*' meaning to join. From a human perspective, the easiest way to understand yoga is to view it as a union of various aspects of the human spirit and body such as the physical, mental, and spiritual being.

In simpler language, we can define yoga as spiritual techniques and exercises that are designed to 'join' your body and mind. It also can help you attain oneness with the universe. Yoga also helps you achieve a healthier lifestyle because it facilitates weight loss, improves blood circulation, and boosts your flexibility.

As we shall see later in the book, different yoga techniques and Asanas demand for specific approaches to derive the expected benefits: unification of various aspects of the human spirit.

In this guide, we shall look at yoga from a varied perspective in a bid to help you derive the benefits offered by yoga.

Before we start discussing how to practice yoga, let us look at the benefits you stand to gain by practicing yoga. By looking at these benefits, you will feel inspired to start your 4-week Yoga challenge.

Why Practice Yoga?

Yoga uses various spiritual and physical exercises that bring many benefits to yoga yogis and yoginis (these are the respective names given to male and female yoga practitioners). For instance, yoga is useful for weight loss, building muscles, relieving stress, and strengthening the heart.

Regular practice can also help you achieve inner peace especially if you pair yoga with meditation. If you are looking for a refreshing leisure activity, yoga can still be an interesting exercise you can practice alone or with friends. Whatever reason you may have for wanting to become a yogi or yogini, yoga can deeply connect your mind, body, and spirit, which can help you experience your real self.

Let us detailedly discuss the various benefits yoga has for its practitioners:

1. Boosts Physical Fitness

Yoga uses various poses and stretches; what we call asanas. Research shows that holding asanas for at least 60 seconds can boost your posture and deadlift strength. Yoga can boost balance of strength onto your opposing muscle groups, and help you improve flexibility and range of motion.

The good thing is that yoga poses are simple and can fit everyone ranging from body builders, athletes, the obese, and members of either gender. When practiced properly, yoga reduces stress buildup in the muscles, relaxes you, and prevents possible workout injuries because it improves flexibility.

To benefit from yoga in terms of strength gains, elongated muscles, and boosting physical fitness, its best to adopt yoga as part of your regular workout program. For instance, doing yoga stretches before strength training allows the muscles to freely workout without actually shutting down in response to stretched tendons.

Better still, yoga aids movement through your full range of motion when hitting weights. With a full range of motion, you can build long and full-toned muscles or abs. Physical fitness experts are of the view that stretching yoga poses elongate the protective heath of connective tissues that cover muscles and its cells and repair worn out muscles.

The main reason why yoga energizes and strengthens muscle groups is the long deep breaths, something you have to do as you practice yoga asanas. These deep breaths supply oxygen to the muscles, and boost your ability to focus on workouts.

Yoga can fit into a busy or sedentary lifestyle. Further, some research shows that yoga can heal chronic pain such as migraines. Without much effort, a beginner yogi such as yourself can learn how to make informed health choices and practice specific yoga asanas and techniques aimed at improving your health. This lifestyle coaching can include various aspects like stress reduction, exercising, diet, mindfulness, and other relaxation techniques.

2. Facilitates Weight Loss

Whichever way you look at it, yoga is both a physical and mental exercise. Research shows that practicing the physical aspect of yoga for around 60 minutes burns around 180-360 calories.

Even with strength training, training experts recommend simple deep breathing and slow poses as one of the ways to tone and effortlessly trim body fat. When you engage in a 90-minute yoga workout session, the deep breathing techniques help heat you up, which flushes out toxins and water weight. This effect boosts the performance of organs as well as the lymphatic system.

Further, specific yoga techniques such as power yoga technique have shown to offer triple benefits such as cardio training, flexibility, and strength training, which facilitates weight-loss.

Unsurprisingly, even the simplest yoga poses have various weight loss benefits because they invoke your hormones, digestion, and breathing control; the three aspects that form the parasympathetic nervous system.

Once activated, the nervous system balances hormones, repairs injuries, and boosts digestion, processes that aid weight loss. For this reason, normal weight and obese yogis are less likely to gain weight when compared to individuals who fail to practice yoga. Furthermore, regular practice of yoga links to mindful eating, improved sleep, and higher rate of self-awareness, factors that help yogis or yoginis lose unwanted weight or maintain healthy body weight effortlessly.

Yoga poses require concentration; this concentration helps dieters eat mindfully. Those who eat mindfully are less likely to overeat and thus less likely to be obese. The increased awareness created by yoga has a weight loss effect and can boost sensitivity to hunger and satiety.

Here, the spiritual and physiology aspects of yoga help dieters eat less compared to the physical aspect of yoga poses. Mindfulness is a technique that yogis can learn directly or indirectly. Mindfulness techniques such as mindful eating have great impact on eating habits. Compared to physical exercises like walking or jogging, Yoga has a strong link to mindfulness. This mindfulness helps dieters determine when they are hungry (instead of binge eating), eat and stop once full.

3. Alleviates Stress

Stress, anxiety, and worries from day-to-day challenges and demanding obligations can cause depression, or worsen symptoms of other mood related diseases. In mild cases, stress causes physical symptoms such as headaches, hypertension, chest pain, stomach upset, sleep problems, or low sexual drive. In extreme cases, stress can lead to emotional problems such as panic attacks, depression, or heart attacks.

Because it refreshes the mind, Yoga can be beneficial as a stress management strategy because when you practice yoga asanas, you relax and tense your muscles; this, coupled with mindfulness techniques helps practitioners develop various physical sensations.

Due to these benefits, yoga actually works to relax your mind and create a calmness you cannot achieve with other workout programs that often leave you feeling exhausted. According to studies, 8 weeks of regular yoga practice can help fight insomnia and improve sleep quality. Relaxation and better sleep can relieve physiological conditions such as clinical depression, calm the mind, and stimulate higher brain functioning. Compared to other cardio exercises such as running or splinting, yoga brings better results without the need to overwork your body.

As you can see, yoga has immense benefits. In the next section, we shall look at how you can adopt yoga as an integral part of your regular exercise routine in 4 weeks.

How to Adopt Yoga in 4 weeks: A Three Step Approach

The key to making yoga work for you is to start with easy and short poses until you accustom to hours of advanced yoga exercises. Further, it is advisable to start training at home before attending professional classes. To do so, consider buying "guided yoga" DVDs, learn basic starter yoga asanas online (you can check on YouTube), and allocate 5-10 minutes to each yoga session.

To make yoga sessions smooth, dedicate a small area of your home house – say a small area of your study room or the floor between the coffee table and the fireplace – as your yoga 'studio.' Whatever setting you choose, ensure it is quiet and free from outside interruption, and comfortable.

Once ready, proceed with these three simple steps:

Step 1: Calm Down

As you begin practicing yoga, you will quickly realize that yoga is not as easy as it may appear. For instance, you may discover your athletic or obese build does not allow for yoga poses that require specific twists or movement.

For basic yoga poses, you need to remain calm and relaxed to facilitate slow and steady progress. Being calm is also a prerequisite to attempting difficult or advanced poses, which like it or not, bring more relief and improved health. If you cannot calm down instantly or at will, try a few breathing exercises such as deep breathing to the count of 4. You can also try warm-up exercises as discussed here.

Step 2: Focus On Your Breath

Breathing is a normal exercise. Unfortunately, most of us do not breathe in a "healthy manner" through the diaphragm – what we call deep breathing. Yoga is all about deep breathing, meditation, physical poses, among other techniques.

For this reason, you need to train yourself to breathe deeply in order to lower cortisol levels and fight stress. When practicing breathing, do it through the nose all through into the belly as detailed in the following steps:

1. Sit on the floor or bed with your legs closed

2. Place the right hand on the bed behind you and then place the left hand on the right knee

3. Sit up straight and deeply breathe for 4-8 counts; as you do, lengthen your spine

4. Begin to exhale; as you twist toward the right, ensure you do not strain the neck

5. Hold this pose for five full breaths, and lengthen the spine on the inhale

6. If you are comfortable with it, deepen the twist on the exhales. If necessary, repeat on the other side.

Deep breathing is an ideal way to meditate before getting into actual yoga; you also may set an intention goal, a prayer, or other objectives at the start of brief meditation.

Step 3: Start With Basic Postures

As a beginner, most yoga poses or stretches could be a big challenge; however, with time and practice, you can master basic and advanced asanas. At this stage of your practice, begin with warm-up poses and then progress to basic yoga poses.

Try a few poses such as the seated twist, forward bend, triangle, cobra, cat, down dog, or mountain. To work out and achieve the yoga benefits detailed earlier, move in all directions simply by selecting a pose for each direction your body moves. This could be twisting, leaning forward or backwards, turning upside down, or leaning side to side. Whatever movement you work on, practice it in all directions to complete your practice.

Once comfortable with these easy poses, you can progress to medium-challenge, or advanced yoga techniques. After each yoga session, end with a relaxation pose. For instance, you can rest on your back and then consciously relax your body for 5-15 minutes. You may then practice short-seated meditation to integrate your yoga practice and get back into your normal daily routine.

How can you become a yoga guru in four weeks? One easy way is progressively adopting different types of yoga techniques from simple warm-up exercises to complicated twists and backbends. For simplicity, this book categorizes yoga poses you can adopt on a week-to-week basis.

Week One

In week one, practice the following yoga asanas:

Warm-Up Exercises

Warm-up exercises are important because they help your mind to safely transition into the yoga practice. As a beginner, you may need to use warm-up poses throughout your yoga session; therefore, do not shy away from doing them this entire week.

Warm-up yoga exercises will open your shoulders muscles, the groin, lower back, the hips, and spine. Here is a whole-body yoga warm-up sequence you can perform as a standalone or combine with other warm-up exercises discussed below.

As you engage in this exercise, ensure to use gentle "fluid movements" that have a perfect blend with slow deep breathing. To realize deeper and effective results, hold each stretch for about 1-2 breaths. However, if you suffer from neck, arms, and back injuries, exercise caution because a failure to do so may exacerbate the problem.

1. The best way is to begin in the easy pose. Here, you should keep your shoulders down and back, the spine elongated, and the chest open.

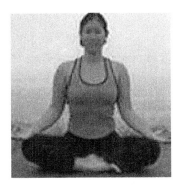

2. Take a deep breath and gently raise the fingertips to the ceiling. With the shoulders down and back, ground the hips to the ground and reach with the fingerprints.

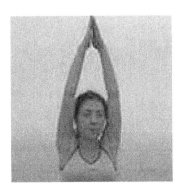

3. At this point, exhale and then round forward with the palms placed on the floor. Round the spine and relax the head and your elbows.

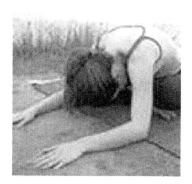

4. Inhale, and raise the fingers up to the ceiling. Keep your shoulders fairly down and back, and the hips firmly grounded to the floor.

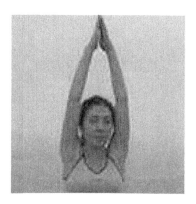

5. Start to exhale as you twist to the left, position the left hand on the right knee and your right hand behind the back. Look over the right shoulder and behind you. Keep the spine elongated and the shoulders down.

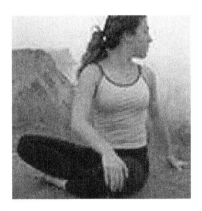

6. Take a deep breath and lift your fingertips up towards the ceiling. Just like before, maintain your shoulders down & back. Moreover, ensure the hips are very much grounded to the floor.

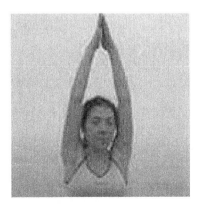

7. Exhale as you twist to the right. Position the right hand onto the left knee and the left hand behind the back. Look over the left shoulder and behind you. The spine should be long and the shoulders down.

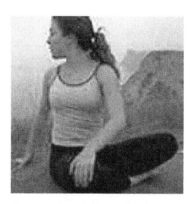

8. Inhale and again, lift the fingertips to the ceiling. Maintain the hips grounded to the floor and the shoulders down and back.

9. This time, exhale and twist the left hand to the floor, and then arch to the left. You should reach out using the right fingers and then lower the left elbow as close to the floor as you can bear. Maintain your chin off the chest and the right arm over your right ear.

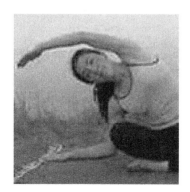

10. With the shoulders down and back, take a deep gentle breath and reach for the ceiling through the fingertips.

11. Breathe out, turn the right hand to the floor, and arch to the right. You should reach through the left fingers and then lower your right elbow closer to the floor as possible. Ensure the chin is off your chest and keep the right arm over the left ear.

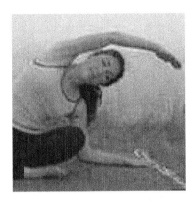

12. Take another deep breath and slowly lift the fingertips up to the ceiling. As you exhale, point the hands forwards and round your spine. Drop the head as you reach out through the fingertips.

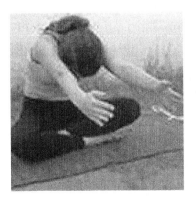

13. Take a deep breath and position the arms behind you. Try to reach back through your fingertips in order to draw the shoulder blades together and then press forward through your chest as you look up.

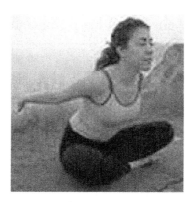

14. Breathe out and place your hands on the knees or the floor. With the shoulders down and back, gently bring the spine back to a neutral position.

15. At this point, you can repeat the warm-up exercise or instead, begin the asana sequences outlined below.

Standing Asanas

Standing yoga asana help align your feet and body because they open the hips, strengthen your back, stretch your legs, and boost your range of movement. Standing yoga poses also bring about various other benefits like facilitating digestion, improving blood circulation, and even aiding weight loss. On top of the physical benefits, a few of standing yoga asanas can have mental and spiritual benefits.

Let us look at a few of such exercises and the benefits you can achieve from them:

1: Mountain pose

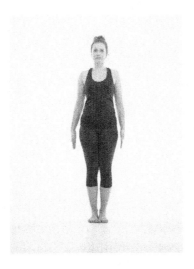

This pose is the foundation of other standing poses. Regularly practicing it can increase your body height and posture. When on this pose, your vertebral column and your heart straighten, while the arms and legs strengthen to fight lethargy. This pose can also promote balance and facilitate focus on the present moment (mindfulness).

To practice the mountain pose, follow these steps:

1. Stand upright and put the feet together ensuring you evenly ground down through the feet.

2. Lift up through the crown of the head.

3. Lift the thighs and then proceed to lengthen up through the 4 sides of the waist. In doing so, elongate the spine and breathe easy.

2: Triangle

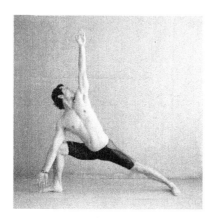

The triangle pose boosts your balance, exercises your inner thighs and hamstrings, and allows your body to expand. With enough practice, you can achieve the flexibility required in this pose.

1. Stand with both feet wide apart then slightly turn-in your left toes to rotate your right thigh open. Then continue until you get the right toes to start pointing directly to the side.

2. Then ground through the feet and then pull the thighs up while keeping your legs fairly straight.

3. Widely spread your arms at shoulder height, then proceed to roll the front thigh open, and then go on to hinge the front side of your hips.

4. Try to lengthen the spine to the direction of the front foot.

3: Warrior One

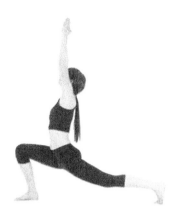

The warrior's pose calms and relieves a troubled mind, boosts stamina, and can strengthen the legs and ankles.

1. Start from a downward-facing dog pose and then step the right foot forward between the hands.

2. Turn the left heel in and as you inhale, lift up the arms and torso. Ensure the heel of your front foot is in line with the back of the back foot's arch.

3. Keep the front of the knee just directly over your ankle, point both the hips forward, and then draw your tailbone down while pulling the ribs in.

4. Make sure your hip's back faces fairly forward and not outward then proceed to turn the back of the feet to around 45 degrees.

5. Repeat the pose on the other side.

4: Half-Moon Pose

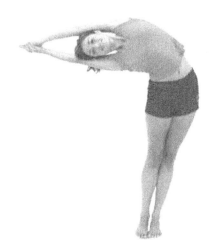

Practicing this pose stretches the sides of the stomach, which strengthens the core and helps burn belly fat. The half-moon pose also tones the upper and inner thighs as well as the buttocks in all genders. To practice, follow these steps:

1. First, stand upright with your feet together. Raise your hands over the head and clasp the palms together. You should extend your stretch by attempting to reach for the ceiling.

2. Breathe out and gradually bend sideways from the hips, as you keep the hands together.

3. Keep the elbows straight without bending forward until you fully experience the "stretch feeling" that comes from the fingertips and thighs.

4. After a few seconds, breathe in and return to the initial standing pose.

5. Repeat the half-moon pose on the other side.

Week Two

In week two, progress to the following asanas:

Note: Remember to practice the warm up and calming asanas as detailed earlier:

Seated and Kneeling Asanas

Seated and kneeling yoga poses help you connect with the breath and offer you calmness and a quiet feeling that revitalizes your entire being and body. Most seated and kneeling yoga asanas help shape your buttocks and legs and, boost spine vitality and flexibility. Below are the several kneeling and seated yoga poses you can practice in week two:

5: Easy Pose

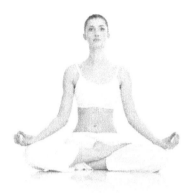

In this meditative yoga asana, you comfortably sit cross-legged on the carpet or ground for a few minutes. This pose allows you to calm down and relieve stress and anxiety in 3-5 minutes. You can also adopt the easy pose for meditation and prayers. To practice, follow these steps:

1. Sit comfortably on a carpet or yoga mat

2. Bend both knees and get into a cross-legged position; ensure your waist, back and neck align in a straight line.

3. Ensure the hands are on your knees; touch the index finger with the tip of the thumb, with the other three fingers straight.

4. Continue to breathe rhythmically for about 5 minutes.

5. If desired, you can increase the duration of your practice to 15 or 30 minutes.

6: Child's Pose

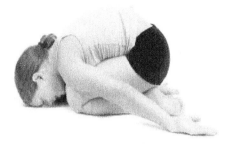

The pose can help you to relax and even enable you to breathe into your back. That's not all; it can help relieve back and neck pains mainly because it usually stretches the thighs, ankles, and hips.

1. Start by sitting upright on your heels then proceed to roll your torso forward

2. Then bring your forehead to rest on the ground just in front of you

3. Then lower your chest to your knees as close as possible and extend the arms backwards or forward.

4. Hold the pose while breathing into the torso

5. Exhale and release while getting deeper into the fold.

7: Half-Split Pose

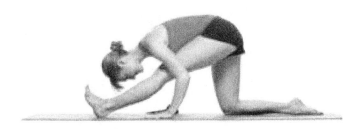

This pose stretches the groin, hamstrings, and thighs and can actually even work as a great workout regime that can help you to achieve tightness in your legs especially if you are an athlete.

1. Get into the Downward-Facing Dog; strongly ground the palms, and then lift the hips up and back.

2. Breathe easy for a few times and then bend the knees. Lift the heels and open up through the back of the legs.

3. As you breathe out, step the right foot forward between the hands, and then lower down onto your left knee; release the upper part of your left foot onto the floor.

4. Then proceed to flex the right foot, to come up to the heel and then extend the toes towards you. Start to straighten the right leg as much as you can manage.

5. Ensure the hips remain square and stacked over the left knee. Breathe easy to facilitate lengthening of the spine and then breathe out as you fold over your right leg.

6. As you reach the chest forward, draw the right heel back and then draw the shoulder blades down your back and from the ears.

7. Maintain the pose for about 5-10 breath, then tuck the left toes under, plant your palms, and get back into the beginning pose.

8. Once ready and relaxed, repeat on the other side

Week Three

In week three, progressively move from last week's asanas into the following ones:

Supine & Prone Asanas

These yoga asanas get rid of any accumulated tension from the abdomen and enhance the mobility of your spine. Supine and prone poses restore strength in your arms, legs, back, and release your hips and groins.

8: Locust Pose

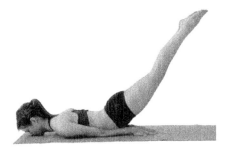

This pose works to relief stress, but can also strengthen muscles in the legs and abdomen.

1. Lie on your belly with the face looking down, and the chin resting gently on the floor.

2. Bring the legs together, and then stretch the leg back with the toes stretching outward.

3. Ensure the pubis firmly presses into the mat and maintain the arms stretched back with the palms up. Be as relaxed as possible.

4. Clench the hands to form fists, and stiffen the arms, legs, and knees.

5. Breathe in slowly to exert a little pressure onto the balled fists and then lift both legs as high as possible: Do not bend the legs.

6. Hold the pose for 15-30 seconds and hold the breath as long as you can bear.

7. As you slowly lower your legs, slowly breathe out.

9: Shoulder Stand

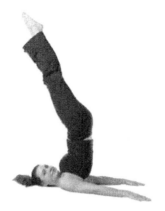

This pose strengthens the entire body; particularly, it strengthens the arm and back muscles.

1. Begin by lying flat on your back and then take a deep breath.

2. Exhale as you lift both legs straight upwards and join them so you can balance your weight on the head, upper arms, shoulders, and neck.

3. Use your hands to support your hips or alternatively, leave the hands flat on the floor.

4. Hold the pose and breathe gently and deeply.

10: Bridge Pose

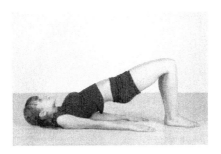

The bridge pose opens your chest and stretches the neck and spine. The pose effectively reduces anxiety, calms the mind, and boosts digestion.

1. Begin at a lying position with your knees bent, arms at sides, and feet flat on the floor.

2. Maintain the feet parallel and hip-width apart. You should stack the heels under the knees.

3. Roll the upper arms open in order to expand your chest. Through the outer upper arms, proceed to ground and then root down into the heels.

4. Continue with this until you reach the knees forward to lift the hips from the ground.

5. Shake your shoulders under the chest and then interlace the fingers.

6. In case you find your shoulders tight, try holding onto the side of the yoga mat. This should help you create more space.

11: Downward Facing Dog Pose

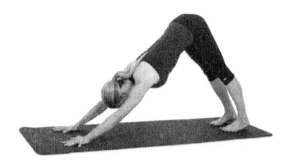

This exercise targets your shoulders, triceps, biceps, and upper body. It also tends to create a fairly calming effect.

1. Start in a plank pose – the up part of a push-up – then bend your elbows as far as possible, and straighten them

2. Lift the hips while you push back into the downward dog pose as you press your heels towards the floor

3. Return to plank pose and repeat this pose 10 times.

Twists Asanas

Twist poses release spine tension, sooth backaches, and align the shoulders and make them more flexible. Twist exercises boost the circulation of blood and other nutrients within the body, which benefits the inter-vertebral discs.

12: Half-Spinal Twist

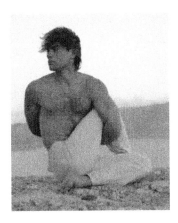

Physical fitness experts believe this yoga pose can boost lungs capacity thus making the lungs capable of handling more oxygen. This asana also tones the abdominal and thigh muscles on top of stretching your spine.

1. With legs stretched out straight in front of you, sit up while keeping the feet together and the spine upright.

2. Bend the left leg and position the heel of the left feet beside the right hip. Alternatively, you can maintain the left leg straight.

3. Position the right leg right over your left knee and then place your left hand onto your right knee while the right hand is right behind you.

4. Proceed to twist at the waist, as well as the shoulders, and the neck following this pattern to your right and then look over the right shoulder.

5. Hold the pose and progress with gentle long breaths in and out.

6. Once done, return to the initial pose, exhale, and release the right hand behind you.

7. Gently release the waist, the chest, the neck, and sit up straight. Repeat on the other side.

13: Seated Twist

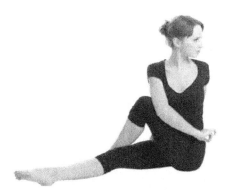

The seated twist is a powerful stretch that you can use after long hours of sitting. It works out the back, hips, and shoulders.

1. Start by sitting on the ground or a carpet with the legs extended

2. Close the right foot over the outside of the left thigh and then bend the left knee.

3. Ensure your right knee is facing towards the ceiling and ensure your right hand is on the ground right behind you. This will stabilize your body.

4. Position the left elbow on the outside of the right knee. Move from your abdomen and Twist to the right as far as possible.

5. Ensure the two sides of your butt are touching the ground.

6. Then repeat the pose on both sides.

14: Low Lunge Twist

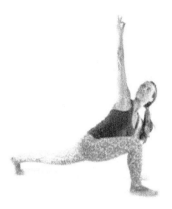

This pose opens the legs, groins, spine, shoulders, and the hips.

1. Start from a downward dog pose.

2. Round your right knee towards your nose and then step the right foot between your hands

3. Release your back knee to the floor.

4. Plant the left palm on the floor in line with the right foot, just under the shoulders.

5. Lift your right arms up towards the roof/sky then take about 3-5 breaths. Once relaxed, repeat the pose on the other side.

Week Four

You are now in the last week of the 4-week yoga challenge. In this week, practice the following asanas:

Inverted and Balance Asana

As the name suggests, these poses defy gravity in order to create coordination, boost your stamina and strength, increase grace, agility and poise. The asanas also boost your focus and concentration because as you practice the asana, you maintain focus and concentration.

15: Tree Pose

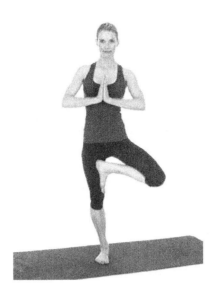

This asana boosts focus and balance; thus, it is an effective way to relieve stress. It strengthens the arches of your feet alongside the outer hips.

1. Begin in the mountain pose and then bend one knee. Using one of your hands, bring the foot into your upper inner thigh.

2. Alternatively, you can try to bring your feet to the shin below your knee, or instead, use a nearby wall for balance.

3. Press into the foot that you are standing on and then lengthen it up through the head's crown.

16: Half Moon

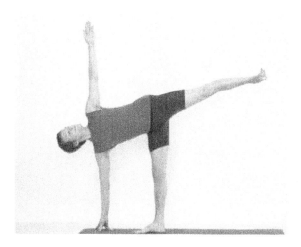

This pose effectively strengthens the outer hips and legs. It stretches the inner thighs and hamstring, and improves your concentration and focus.

1. Begin in the triangle pose

2. Bend the front knee as you track it using the second toe

3. Step up the back foot in and then walk your bottom hand about 12 inches in front of you.

4. Using the pinky toe, line up your thumb and shift your entire weight onto the front foot. Lift the back foot from the floor.

5. Strongly reach the back leg to the direction of the wall behind you as you raise up the top arm.

6. Rotate the chest to the ceiling in order to challenge your balance, and then gaze up at your top hand.

17: Crow Pose

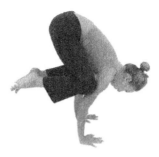

This pose strengthens the abs, arms, and wrists.

1. Start in the downward facing dog pose and then walk the feet forward in order for the knees to touch the arms.

2. Proceed to bend the elbows carefully while lifting your heels from the ground. Then position your knees against the outside of your upper arms

3. Keep your legs fairly pressed against your arms and your abs fairly engaged.

4. You can also place the toes on the floor or instead, lift them off and over. Ensure you keep tucked tight and place the heels very close to the butt.

5. Once you are ready, proceed to push your upper arms right against your shins and then proceed to draw the inner groins very deep into your pelvis in order to facilitate the lift.

18: Eagle Pose

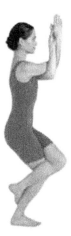

The eagle pose aids focus or concentration by enhancing balance and coordination.

1. Stand in a mountain pose and then slightly bend your knees. As you balance on your right foot, lift the left foot up and cross the left thigh over the right.

2. Ensure your left toes are facing the floor and then press the foot back. Hook the very top of your foot just behind your lower calf and then try to balance on your right foot.

3. Stretch the arms forward, parallel to the floor, and move the scapulas to spread wide across the back of the torso.

4. Cross the arm in front of the torso so that the right arm is above the left and then bend the elbows.

5. Tightly fit the right elbow into the crook of the left, and then lift your forearms to form a right angle in respect to the floor. Ensure the back of the hands face each other.

6. Then proceed to press your right hand to the right alongside your left hand to your left. Here, you should make your palms to face each other, while the right hand's thumb is passing in front of your left hand's little finger.

7. From this pose, press the palms together as much as you can bear and then lift the elbows. Next, stretch the fingers to the direction of the ceiling.

8. Maintain the pose for about 15-30 seconds and then unwind your arms as well as legs to get into the mountain pose.

9. Reverse the arms and legs and repeat a couple of times.

Conclusion

By practicing yoga every day for 4 weeks, the practice will become a habit and within no time, you will be a master yogi who can perform even the most advanced asanas. As you practice the asanas outlined in this guide, remember to stay safe and avoid injury as much as you possibly can.

I hope this book was able to help you to understand how you can incorporate yoga into your life in as little as 4 weeks.

The next step is to implement what you have learnt.

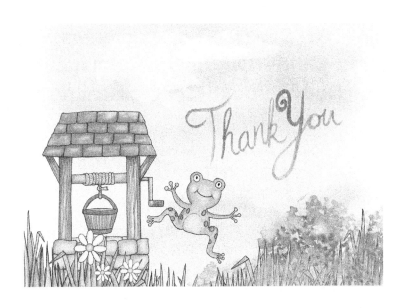

Finally, if you enjoyed this book, then Id like to ask you for a favor, would you be kind enough to leave a review for this book on Amazon?

Thank you and good luck!

Preview Of 'Chakras For Beginners: The 7 Chakras Guide On How to Balance your Energy Body through Chakra Healing'

Introduction

Have you heard about Chakras but aren't sure what they are and how they can improve your life? The fact is that Chakras are energy points located throughout the body. When one of points becomes blocked, energy cannot flow as it is intended to flow. Thus, there are certain actions that you can take to heal the flow and make sure that the Chakra is cleared.

This book assumes that you are a beginner. It explores where the Chakras are located and what each one of them does to your sense of wellbeing. When you learn that, you also learn to respect your posture, your interaction with others, and increase your self-esteem levels by making sure that the Chakras are always in perfect alignment.

Although you may be a little doubtful about whether this really works, it has been proven over centuries and is not something new. Those who have been able to keep the Chakras open to the flow of energy that life offers them, tend to be healthy and happy. This book is written to help you to achieve that same level of happiness that is available for all, but that few achieve because of their own inadequacies.

Chapter 1 – The Location of the Chakras

Ever felt pain and pressure in the back of your neck? The chances are that you are stressed and that the chakra, located in the neck region, is taking on all of that negative energy. Negative energy stops you in your tracks and can really make life difficult. This chakra is probably one of the most obvious in the body even to those who know little about the Chakra system. However, do you know where the other Chakras are located? Chances are that you don't. In this chapter, we make you aware of them so that you know from your own experiences that Chakra is giving you problems.

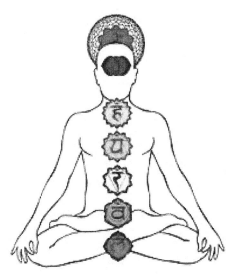

1. The Crown Chakra

2. The Third Eye Chakra

3. The Throat Chakra

4. The Heart Chakra

5. The Solar Plexus Chakra

6. The Sacral Chakra

7. The Base/Root Chakra

The crown chakra is located at the top of the head. The Third Eye chakra is located between the lines of your eyebrows. The throat chakra placement is obvious. The heart Chakra is located in the center of your body at heart level. The Sacral Chakra is just below your tummy button, while your solar plexus chakra is about 3 inches above the tummy button. The base chakra is located at the base of the spine.

You can see that these are represented by colors and symbols each of which have meaning. However, as a beginner, it's more important that you know which kind of problems relate to each of the Chakras, so that you can perform the exercises or activities needed to open up that Chakra in times of need. Let's run through the kind of things that each of these Chakras is responsible for, so that you gain a better understanding. It is not as complex as acupuncture because in acupuncture, there are many pressure points. Thus learning about the Chakras is much easier for the beginner than learning other systems of energy control.

The Crown Chakra – If the Crown Chakra is out of whack, you may be experiencing depression. You may also have problems with your concentration. Any mental blockage of any kind can come from this region. In fact, if you are short tempered because of sounds or the density of light, perhaps it is this Chakra that is out of alignment. In a later chapter, we will talk about balancing the chakra responsible for your lack of alignment, though for now, we merely discuss the illnesses likely to be caused by a blockage in a certain chakra.

The Third Eye Chakra – This is responsible for all kinds of things, including blurred vision, lack of intuitive thought, hearing loss, sinus problems etc., but it doesn't stop there. If you have emotional problems then this Chakra is like to play a part. If you feel the need to exaggerate to gain the attention of others, then this is a weakness that could be accounted for by the blockage of this Chakra.

The Throat Chakra – As we already explained stress can cause this chakra to be blocked, but there are other health issues as well. For example, Thyroid conditions, facial pain or even ear infections can all be caused by the blockage of this particular chakra.

The Heart Chakra – This is an important Chakra when it comes to illnesses that are serious. Lung disease, heart problems and pains in the lower arm can all be attributable to a blockage of this chakra. If you find that your upper back area has problems or your shoulders hurt, this is also likely to be the chakra that is causing that pain. Emotional imbalances may be the cause of this Chakra being out of alignment too and this includes feelings of jealousy, insecurity with relationships or any anger that comes from your relationships with others.

The Solar Plexus Chakra – This chakra is related to digestive problems, gall bladder problems and even chronic fatigue. That feeling of butterflies in the stomach or nervousness when faced by new things comes from this region as well as fears of being rejected.

The Sacral Chakra – If you suffer from urinary problems, this is likely to be the offender. Pains that arise in the lower back area can also come from this chakra, as can liver problems. This chakra is a great chakra to balance because it gives you dynamism and confidence.

The Root Chakra – This accounts for problems below the area where the chakra is located and that can include knee problems, immunity problems, prostate gland problems, sciatica and even illnesses such as constipation or ailments caused by eating disorders. The root chakra also acts as the main chakra to take account of people's feelings of having all of their needs in life fulfilled, such as housing or being able to support oneself. This chakra is likely to be blocked when your living situation feels out of control.

As you can see, we have generalized each of the areas of the Chakras so that you get a clue as to which Chakra is blocked, depending upon the difficulty that you are currently encountering.

Look inside ⇩

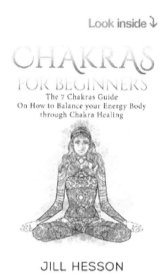

CHAKRAS
FOR BEGINNERS
The 7 Chakras Guide
On How to Balance your Energy Body
through Chakra Healing

JILL HESSON

http://amzn.to/2bDA6xf

Here Is A Preview Of What You Can Learn From This Book.

- The Location of the Chakras
- Changing your Lifestyle for the Better
- Healing of the Chakras
- Healing the Throat Chakra
- Yoga Poses for the Other Chakras
- And Much More

Check out the rest of the book by searching for this title on Amazon website.

CPSIA information can be obtained
at www.ICGtesting.com
Printed in the USA
BVOW06s1823260617

487867BV00018B/129/P